The Ultimate Keto Diet Recipe Book 2021

A Keto-Friendly Recipe Compilation to Lose Weight Guilt-Free

Camilla Ingram

TABLE OF CONTENTS

INTRODUCTION		5
BREAKFAST		9
1.	Broccoli and Cheese Squash	9
2.	Butter Garlic Spinach	11
3.	Crock Pot Muffin Casserole	12
4.	Crestless Crock Pot Spinach Quiche	14
5.	Scrambled Eggs with Smoked Salmon	15
6.	Garlic-Parmesan Asparagus Crock Pot	17
7.	Persian Omelet Crock Pot	18
LUNCH		20
8.	Mashed Turnips	20
9.	Cilantro Meatballs	22
10.	Stuffed Jalapenos	23
11.	BBQ Beef Short Ribs	24
12.	Spiced Beef	25
13.	Green Peas Chowder	26
14.	Zucchini Pasta	27
15.	Chinese Broccoli	28
16.	Slow Cooker Spaghetti Squash	29
17.	Mushroom Stew	30
DINNER		32
18.	Chicken & Kale Soup	32
19.	Chicken Chili Soup	34
20.	Creamy Smoked Salmon Soup	36
21.	Lamb and Rosemary Stew	38
22.	Pork Shoulder with Noodles	39
23.	Teriyaki Pork with Tortillas	41
24.	Pork Chops with Creamy Sauce	42
25.	Pork Chops with Apricot and Hoisin Sauce	44
26.	Pork Chops with Honey and Mustard	45

27.	Smoked Pork with Prunes	46
28.	Sweet Orange Smoked Ham	48
29.	Sherry Chicken with Mashed Potatoes	49

SNACKS RECIPES — 52

30.	Nectarines with Dried Cloves	52
31.	Chocolate Raspberry Parfait	53
32.	Patbingsu – In Moderation	56

VEGETABLE RECIPES — 59

33.	Cheese Stuffed Spaghetti Squash	59
34.	Cottage Kale Stir-Fry	61
35.	Herbed Eggplant and Kale Bake	62

POULTRY RECIPES — 65

36.	Chicken Meatloaf Cups with Pancetta	65
37.	Turkey Wing Curry	67
38.	Double-Cheese Ranch Chicken	69
39.	Turkey and Canadian Bacon Pizza	71

FISH AND SEAFOOD RECIPES — 73

40.	Coconut Mussels	73
41.	Italian Style Halibut Packets	75
42.	Hazelnut Haddock Bake	78
43.	Coconut and Pecorino Fried Shrimp	80
44.	Greek Tilapia with Tomatoes and Olives	82

SALAD RECIPES — 84

| 45. | Charred Broccoli and Sardine Salad | 84 |
| 46. | Zucchini and Bell Pepper Slaw | 85 |

DESSERT — 87

47.	Delicious Peach Crisp	87
48.	Gingerbread Pudding Cake	88
49.	Healthy Blueberry Cobbler	90
50.	Easy Peach Cobbler	91

KETO MEDITERRANEAN RECIPES — 92

| 51. | Vanilla Frozen Yogurt | 92 |

52.	Chia Berry Yogurt Parfaits	94
53.	Lemon Meringue Cookies	96
54.	Strawberry Cheesecake Jars	98
55.	Tuscan Garlic Chicken	100
56.	Garlic & Rosemary Lamb Lollipops	102
57.	Greek Chicken	103
58.	Lemon Chicken	105
59.	Chicken Pesto Meatballs	107
60.	Parmesan Chicken	109

INTRODUCTION

The ketogenic diet, abbreviated as keto, is a low-carbohydrate diet that is associated with people seeking fast and drastic weight loss. For certain people, losing weight has become a no-brainer - a weight-loss diet that requires a high-fat, low-carbohydrate diet in addition to a nutritious diet of fruits and vegetables. Although a diet high in carbohydrates - fats, low in carbohydrates - can help alleviate appetite and increase weight loss, the "keto diet" is not a true thing.

According to research, a high-fat diet has a detrimental effect on cholesterol and triglycerides, even though carbohydrate consumption stays extremely poor. There is now proof that the keto diet, which is low in fat but high in starch and fat, will help you survive longer than a low-fat diet.

In this case, the body requires less carbs and can perform best on a low-carbohydrate diet such as Atkins, which can be taxing on your kidneys. To enter ketosis, you must limit your calorie intake in order to lose weight on the keto diet.

Keto dieters should stick to keto diets that include fiber-rich foods such as bananas, vegetables, whole grains, nuts, and seeds. To get the best out of the keto diet, you need to concentrate on more than just meeting one of the "keto macros." Concentrate on a ketogenic diet and improving your diet's sustainability, and you'll be able to concentrate on your physical health and well-being rather than on your weight loss goals.

Individuals who adopt a ketogenic diet resist some fruits and vegetables due to their high carbohydrate content. Reducing carbohydrate consumption, like certain individuals do in ketosis, entails a reduction of protein intake, which health advocates condemn. Since brain deterioration and illness have distinct etiologies, you will be able to use either a low-carb or a high-carb diet - or a combination of the two - to treat and reduce the danger.

If you are on a low-carb diet on a daily basis, particularly over an extended period of time, you might consider switching to a carbohydrate diet. Nowadays, experts often believe that you should follow a ketogenic diet indefinitely if your weight is within a safe range and your blood values are within a normal range. If you are committed to avoiding ketosis in the long run, the doctor would almost always recommend that you take vitamins and supplements to ensure that you have all of the nutrients you need to remain healthy. For newcomers, the ketone diet's fundamentals can be shockingly simple to adopt, especially though you are new to this sort of diet plan.

The keto diet is protein-restricted, with extra calories converted to glucose to induce ketosis. It is comparable to the Atkins and Paleo diets in that it places a greater emphasis on fat intake even though protein is not consumed.

Although the protein and decreasing carbohydrate intake are the most popular modifications to the keto diet, they may result in health problems. This results in weight gain and the resulting health complications including elevated blood pressure, diabetes, heart disease, and high cholesterol.

As a result, I would still warn against fad diets, such as the brief ketogenic diet. Weight reduction is a temporary gain, and the long-term health advantages of a ketogenic diet, which is low in carbs and high in fat, are difficult to sustain, according to the American Heart Association.

The ketogenic diet, abbreviated keto, is a low-fat, high-carbohydrate diet that has been shown to have a variety of health benefits. It is usually considered safe and effective for adults as a short-term nutritional approach, although it does have certain health risks. The following are some foods that are keto-friendly and some that you can stop if you wish to give the ketogenic diet a shot. While a ketogenic diet can be healthier in the short term, it may pose significant health issues in the long run.

However, before we answer these concerns, let us begin with a brief primer: The traditional keto diet is a low-carbohydrate, high-nutrition diet with a high protein, carbohydrate, and fat intake.

The keto diet induces ketosis in the body by consuming diets that are rich in fat and low in carbohydrates. Adhering to the ketosis diet induces a "state of ketosis," which looks similar to ketoacidosis, but is mostly a low-carbohydrate diet. Since too many people who attempt it casually do not track their ketones, they may not be in this condition, or "ketosis."

The Keto diet has been shown in studies to provide amazing, fast weight loss outcomes, at least in the short term. When the benefits and drawbacks of the Keto diet are weighed, it becomes clear that it will potentially be more filling than most diets. I believe it is fair to conclude that an abundance of data shows that this is useful for some individuals for a brief period of time. This means that following a ketogenic diet for an extended period of time may increase your risk of cardiovascular disease and high cholesterol if you do not eat the right foods.

BREAKFAST

1. Broccoli and Cheese Squash

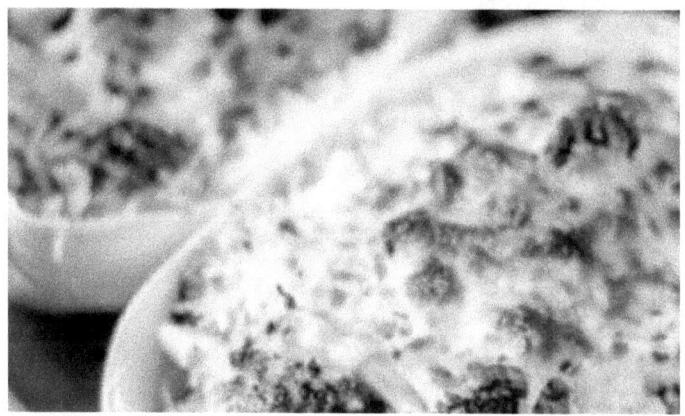

Preparation time: 15 minutes

Cooking time: 3 hours

Servings: 7

Ingredients:

- Squash 1 pcs, halves
- Broccoli florets 2 cups
- Garlic 3 pcs
- Red pepper flakes 1 teaspoon
- Italian season 1 teaspoon
- Mozzarella cheese 1/2 cup
- Parmesan cheese 1/3 cup
- Cooking spray
- Salt and pepper at will

Directions:

1. Set the squash halves in a cooker.
2. Add a little bit of water.
3. .
4. Combine broccoli, minced garlic to the skillet, stir, until the broccoli is tender.
5. Take the squash take off the flesh of the squash. Combine with the broccoli mixture.
6. Cover and cook on low. Serve.

Nutrition: Calories: 230 Carbs: 22g Fat: 5 g Protein: 21g

2. Butter Garlic Spinach

Preparation time: 15 minutes

Cooking time: 1 hour

Servings: 4

Ingredients:

- salted butter 2 tablespoons
- garlic, minced 4 cloves
- Baby spinach 8 oz.
- Pinch of salt
- lemon juice 1 teaspoons

Directions:

1. Dissolve the butter. Sautee the garlic until a bit tender.
2. Put the spinach into the Cooker, combine with salt and lemon juice, tender garlic, butter.
3. Put to cook on low. Brush with fresh lemon wedges. Serve hot.

Nutrition: Calories: 38 Carbs: 2gFat: 3g Protein: 2g

3. Crock Pot Muffin Casserole

Preparation time: 15 minutes

Cooking time: 4 hours

Servings: 7

Ingredients:

- English muffin 1 large, cut into portions
- Canadian bacon1 lb. thick-cut
- eggs 10 large
- milk 1 cup
- salt and pepper
- egg 6 yolks
- lemon juice 1 1/2 tablespoon
- unsalted butter, melted1 1/2 sticks
- salt
- pinch of cayenne

Directions:

1. Dissolve the butter. Combine coconut and almond flour, egg, salt, and stir everything well. Add baking soda.
2. Set the muffin into equal pieces, put on the bottom.
3. Cut the bacon, sprinkle half of it over top of the muffin pieces.
4. Cook on low. Detach, and keep the muffins covered before serving.
5. Whisk carefully; the bowl mustn't get too hot.
6. Season with salt and pepper.

7. Serve and enjoy.
8. Serve and enjoy.

Nutrition: Calories: 286 Carbs: 1.6g Fat: 19g Protein: 14g

4. Crestless Crock Pot Spinach Quiche

Preparation time: 15 minutes

Cooking time: 2 hours

Servings: 11

Ingredients:
- Frozen spinach10 oz. package
- Butter or ghee1 tablespoon
- Red bell pepper1 medium
- Cheddar cheese1 1/2 cups
- Eggs8 pcs
- Homemade sour cream1 cup
- Fresh chives2 tablespoons
- Sea salt1/2 teaspoon
- Ground black pepper1/4 teaspoon
- Ground almond flour 1/2 cup
- Baking soda1/4 teaspoon

Directions:
1. Let the frozen spinach thaw and drain it well. Chop finely. Wash the pepper and slice it. Remove the seeds.
2. Grate the cheddar cheese and set aside. Chop the fresh chives finely.
3. Grease the slow cooker with cooking spray.
4. Attach the almond flour with baking soda.
5. Pour it egg mixture and stir.
6. Set to cook on high

Nutrition: Calories: 153 Carbs: 1.9g Fat: 3g Protein: 9g

5. Scrambled Eggs with Smoked Salmon

Preparation time: 15 minutes

Cooking time: 2 hours

Servings: 6

Ingredients:

- Smoked salmon 1/4 lb.
- eggs12 pcs fresh
- heavy cream1/2 cup
- almond flour1/4 cup
- Salt and black pepper at will
- Butter2 tablespoons
- fresh chives at will

Directions:

1. Cut the slices of salmon. Set aside for garnish. Chop the rest of the salmon into small pieces.
2. Take a medium bowl, whisk the eggs and cream together. Add half of the chopped chives, season eggs with salt and pepper. Add flour.
3. Dissolve the butter over medium heat, then pour into the mixture. Grease the Slow Cooker with oil or cooking spray.
4. Add salmon pieces to the mixture, pour it into the Slow Cooker. Set to cook on low within 2 hours.
5. Garnish the dish with remaining salmon, chives. Serve warm and enjoy!

Nutrition: Calories: 325 Carbohydrate: 5 g Protein: 54 g Fat: 21 g Sugar: 3.4 g Sodium: 1422 mg Fiber: 13.9 g

6. Garlic-Parmesan Asparagus Crock Pot

Preparation time: 15 minutes

Cooking time: 1 hour

Servings: 6

Ingredients:

- olive oil extra virgin 2 tablespoons
- minced garlic 2 teaspoons
- egg 1 pcs fresh
- garlic salt 1/2 teaspoon
- fresh asparagus 12 ounces
- Parmesan cheese 1/3 cup
- Pepper at will

Directions:

1. Peel the garlic and mince it. Wash the asparagus. Shred the Parmesan cheese.
2. Take a medium-sized bowl combine oil, garlic, cracked egg, and salt together. Whisk everything well.
3. Cover the green beans and coat them well.
4. Spread the cooking spray over the Slow Cooker's bottom, put the coated asparagus, season with the shredded cheese. Toss.
5. Cook on high within 1 hour. Once the time is over, you may also season with the rest of the cheese. Serve.

Nutrition: Calories: 132 Carbohydrate: 2.1 g Protein: 32 g Fat: 21 g Sugar: 2.4 g Sodium: 134 mg Fiber: 13.9 g

7. Persian Omelet Crock Pot

Preparation time: 15 minutes

Cooking time: 3 hours

Servings: 14

Ingredients:

- olive oil 2 tablespoons
- butter 1 tablespoons
- red onion 1 large
- green onions 4 pcs
- garlic 2 cloves
- Spinach 2 oz.
- fresh chives 1/4 cup
- cilantro leaves 1/4 cup
- parsley leaves 1/4 cup
- fresh dill 2 tablespoons
- Kosher salt and black pepper at will
- pine nuts 1/4 cup
- eggs 9 large - whole milk 1/4 cup
- Greek yogurt 1 cup

Directions:

1. Take a saucepan to melt the butter. Add red onion, stirring occasionally; it takes about 8-9 minutes.
2. Add green onions, garlic, continue cooking for 4 minutes. Put the spinach, chives, parsley, and cilantro, add salt and pepper at will. Remove the skillet, add the pine nuts.

3. Take a bowl, crack the eggs, add milk, and a little pepper and whisk. Mix the eggs with veggie mixture.
4. Open the Slow Cooker and spread the cooking spray over the bottom and sides. Pour the mix into the Slow Cooker. Cook on low for 3 hours. Serve with Greek yogurt. Bon Appetite!

Nutrition: Calories: 327 Carbohydrate: 3.5 g Protein: 32 g Fat: 13 g Sugar: 13.4 g Sodium: 546 mg Fiber: 11.9 g

LUNCH

8. Mashed Turnips

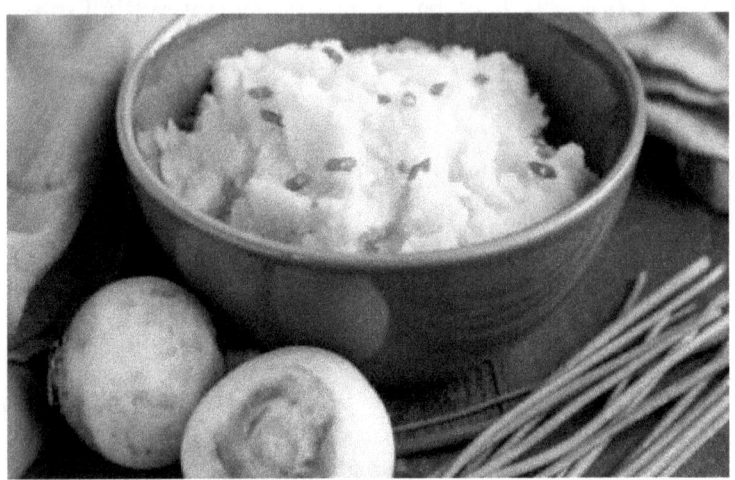

Preparation time: 10 minutes

Cooking time: 7 hours

Servings: 6

Ingredients:

- 3-pounds turnip, chopped
- 2 cup water
- 1tablespoon vegan butter
- 1 tablespoon chives, chopped
- 1oz. Parmesan, grated
- Put turnips in the slow cooker.

Directions

1. Add water and cook the vegetables on low for 7 hours. Then drain water and mash the turnips.

2. Add chives, butter, and Parmesan.
3. Carefully stir the mixture until butter and Parmesan are melted Then add chives. Mix the mashed turnips again.

Nutrition: Calories 198 Fat 19 g Carbohydrates 1.9 g Sugar 3 g Protein 12

9. Cilantro Meatballs

Preparation time: 20 minutes

Cooking time: 4 hours

Servings: 6

Ingredients:
- 1-pound minced beef
- 1 teaspoon minced garlic
- 1 egg, beaten
- 1teaspoon chili flakes
- 2teaspoons dried cilantro
- 1 tablespoon semolina
- 1/2 cup of water
- 1tablespoon sesame oil

Directions
1. In the bowl, mix minced beef, garlic, egg, chili flakes, cilantro, and semolina.
2. Then make the meatballs.
3. After this, heat the sesame oil in the skillet.
4. Cook the meatballs in the hot oil on high heat for 1 minute per side.
5. Transfer the roasted meatballs to the slow cooker, add water, and close the lid.
6. Cook the meatballs on High for 4 hours.

Nutrition: Calories 125 Fat 1 g Carbohydrates 3 g Sugar 3 g Protein 12

10. Stuffed Jalapenos

Preparation time: 10 minutes

Cooking time: 4 hours

Servings: 3

Ingredients:

- 1jalapenos, deseed
- 1oz. minced beef
- 1 teaspoon garlic powder
- 1/2 cup of water

Directions

1. Mix the minced beef with garlic powder.
2. Then fill the jalapenos with minced meat and arrange it in the slow cooker. Add water and cook the jalapenos on High for 4.5 hours.

Nutrition: Calories 154 Fat 3 g Carbohydrates 5 g Sugar 2 g Protein 15

11. BBQ Beef Short Ribs

Preparation time: 10 minutes

Cooking time: 5 hours

Servings: 4

Ingredients:

- 1-pound beef short ribs
- 1/3 cup BBQ sauce
- 1/4 cup of water
- 1 teaspoon chili powder

Directions

1. Rub the beef short ribs with chili powder and put in the slow cooker Mix water with BBQ sauce and pour the liquid into the slow cooker. Cook the meat on High for 5 hours.

Nutrition: Calories 187 Fat 2 g Carbohydrates 1 g Sugar 4 g Protein 21

12. Spiced Beef

Preparation time: 10 minutes

Cooking time: 9 hours

Servings: 4

Ingredients:

- 1-pound beef loin
- 1 teaspoon allspice
- 1 teaspoon olive oil
- 1 tablespoon minced onion
- 1 cup of water

Directions

1. Rub the beef loin with allspice, olive oil, and minced onion.
2. Put the meat in the slow cooker.
3. Add water and close the lid.
4. Cook the beef on Low for 9 hours.
5. When the meat is cooked, slice it into servings.

Nutrition: Calories 187 Fat 2 g Carbohydrates 1 g Sugar 4 g Protein 21

13. Green Peas Chowder

Preparation time: 10 minutes

Cooking time: 8 hours

Servings: 6

Ingredients:

- 1-pound chicken breast, skinless, boneless, chopped
- 2cups water
- 1cup green peas
- 1/4cup Greek Yogurt 1 tablespoon dried basil
- teaspoon ground black pepper 1/2 teaspoon salt

Directions

1. Mix salt, chicken breast, ground black pepper, and dried basil.
2. Transfer the ingredients to the slow cooker.
3. Add water, green peas, yogurt, and close the lid.
4. Cook the chowder on Low for 8 hours.

Nutrition: Calories 213 Fat 3 g Carbohydrates 4 g Sugar 2 g Protein 13

14. Zucchini Pasta

Preparation time: 15 minutes

Cooking time: 1 hour

Servings: 4

Ingredients:

- 2 zucchinis
- 1 teaspoon dried oregano
- 1 teaspoon dried basil
- 2 tablespoons butter
- 1/4 teaspoon salt
- 5 tablespoons water

Directions:

1. Peel the zucchini and spiralize it with a veggie spiralizer.
2. Melt the butter and mix it together with the dried oregano, dried basil, salt, and water.
3. Place the spiralized zucchini in the slow cooker and add the spice mixture.
4. Close the lid and cook the meal for 1 hour on Low.
5. Let the cooked pasta cool slightly.
6. Serve it!

Nutrition: Calories 68, Fat 6, Fiber 1.2, Carbs 3.5, Protein 1.3

15. Chinese Broccoli

Preparation time: 15 minutes

Cooking time: 1 hour

Servings: 4

Ingredients:

- 1 tablespoon sesame seeds
- 1 tablespoon olive oil
- 10 oz. broccoli
- 1 teaspoon chili flakes
- 1 tablespoon apple cider vinegar
- 3 tablespoons water
- 1/4 teaspoon garlic powder

Directions:

1. Cut the broccoli into the florets and sprinkle with the olive oil, chili flakes, apple cider vinegar, and garlic powder.
2. Stir the broccoli and place it in the slow cooker.
3. Add water and sesame seeds.
4. Cook the broccoli for 1 hour on High.
5. Transfer the cooked broccoli to serving plates and enjoy!

Nutrition: Calories 69, Fat 4.9, Fiber 2.1, Carbs 5 Protein 2.4

16. Slow Cooker Spaghetti Squash

Preparation time: 15 minutes

Cooking time: 4 hours

Servings: 5

Ingredients:

- 1-pound spaghetti squash
- 1 tablespoon butter
- 1/4 cup water
- 1 teaspoon ground black pepper
- 1/4 teaspoon ground nutmeg

Directions:

1. Peel the spaghetti squash and sprinkle it with the ground black pepper and ground nutmeg.
2. Pour water in the slow cooker.
3. Add butter and spaghetti squash.
4. Close the lid and cook for 4 hours on Low.
5. Chop the spaghetti squash into small pieces and serve!

Nutrition: Calories 50, Fat 2.9, Fiber 6.6, Carbs 0.1, Protein 0.7

17. Mushroom Stew

Preparation time: 15 minutes

Cooking time: 6 hours

Servings: 8

Ingredients:

- 10 oz. white mushrooms, sliced
- 2 eggplants, chopped
- 1 onion, diced
- 1 garlic clove, diced
- 2 bell peppers, chopped
- 1 cup water
- 1 tablespoon butter
- 1/2 teaspoon salt
- 1/2 teaspoon ground black pepper

Directions:

1. Place the sliced mushrooms, chopped eggplant, and diced onion into the slow cooker.
2. Add garlic clove and bell peppers.
3. Sprinkle the vegetables with salt and ground black pepper.
4. Add butter and water and stir it gently with a wooden spatula.
5. Close the lid and cook the stew for 6 hours on Low.
6. Stir the cooked stew one more time and serve!

Nutrition: Calories 71Fat 1.9, Fiber 5.9, Carbs 1.3, Protein 3

DINNER

18. Chicken & Kale Soup

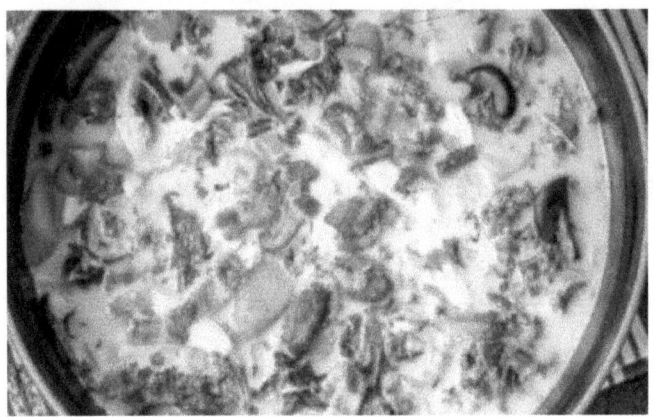

Preparation Time: 5 minutes

Cooking time: 6 hrs.

Servings: 6

Ingredients

- Chicken breast or thigh meat – 2 lbs., without bone or skin
- Chicken broth – 14 oz.
- Olive oil – 1/2 cup, plus 1 tbsp.
- Diced onion – 1/3 cup
- Chicken stock – 32 oz.
- Baby kale leaves – 5 oz.
- Salt and pepper to taste
- Lemon juice – 1/4 cup

Directions:

1. Heat 1 tbsp. of oil in a pan over medium heat.
2. Season the chicken with salt and pepper and place it in the pan.
3. Lower the heat to medium and cover. Cook for 15 minutes or until chicken reaches 165F. Shred the meat and add it to the Crock-Pot.
4. In a bowl, combine the rest of the oil, onion, and chicken broth. Add it to the Crock-Pot.
5. Add the rest of the ingredients and cover.
6. Cook on low for 6 hours. Stir a couple of times as it cooks.

Nutrition: Calories: 261 Fat: 21g Carbs: 2g Protein: 14.1g

19. Chicken Chili Soup

Preparation Time: 5 minutes

Cooking time: 6 hrs.

Servings: 4

Ingredients

- Onion – 1/2, chopped
- Unsalted butter – 1 tbsp.
- Green pepper – 1/2, chopped
- Chicken thighs – 4, boneless
- Bacon – 4 slices
- Salt and pepper to taste
- Thyme – 1/2 tbsp.
- Minced garlic – 1/2 tbsp.
- Coconut flour – 1/2 tbsp.
- Lemon juice – 1 1/2 tbsp.
- Chicken stock – 1/2 cup
- Tomato paste – 1 1/2 tbsp.
- Unsweetened coconut milk – 2 tbsp.

Directions:

1. Add the butter into the Crock-Pot.
2. Add the sliced onion and peppers.
3. Then add the chicken on top, and sprinkle with sliced bacon.
4. Add all the dry ingredients and lastly add the liquids.
5. Cover and cook on low for 6 hours.
6. Mix and break apart the chicken.

7. Serve.

Nutrition: Calories: 396 Fat: 21g Carbs: 5g Protein: 41g

20. Creamy Smoked Salmon Soup

Preparation Time: 5 minutes

Cooking time: 3 hrs.

Servings: 4

Ingredients

- Smoked salmon – 1/2 lb., roughly chopped
- Garlic – 3 cloves, crushed
- Small onion – 1, finely chopped
- Leek – 1, finely chopped
- Heavy cream – 1 1/2 cups
- Olive oil – 2 tbsp.
- Salt and pepper to taste
- Fish stock – 1 1/2 cups

Directions:

1. Add oil into the Crock-Pot.
2. Add fish stock, leek, salmon, garlic, and onion into the pot.
3. Cover with the lid and cook on low for 2 hours.
4. Add the cream and stir. Cook for 1 hour more.
5. Adjust seasoning and serve.

Nutrition: Calories: 309 Fat: 26.4g Carbs: 5g Protein: 12.3g

21. Lamb and Rosemary Stew

Preparation Time: 5 minutes

Cooking time: 8 hrs.

Servings: 4

Ingredients

- Boneless lamb – 1 1/2 lbs., cut into cubes
- Onion – 1, roughly chopped
- Garlic – 3 cloves, finely chopped
- Dried rosemary – 1 tsp.
- Lamb stock cube – 1
- Olive oil – 3 tbsp. divided
- Water – 2 cups
- Salt and pepper to taste

Directions:

1. Add olive oil into the Crock-Pot.
2. Brown the lamb in an oiled skillet for 2 minutes.
3. Add 2 cups of water, stock cube, rosemary, garlic, onion, lamb, salt, and pepper to the pot.
4. Cover with the lid and cook on low for 8 hours.
5. Serve.

Nutrition: Calories: 427 Fat: 23.3g Carbs: 3.9g Protein: 48.6g

22. Pork Shoulder with Noodles

Preparation Time: 5 minutes

Cooking time: 8 hrs.

Servings: 6

Ingredients

- pork shoulder roast, boneless
- 1 cup red onion, chopped
- 1 cup chicken broth
- 1/4 cup dry cherry
- 1 teaspoon garlic powder
- 1 teaspoon celery seeds
- 1/2 teaspoon cumin seeds
- Sea salt, to taste
- Ground black pepper, to taste
- tablespoons cornstarch
- 1/3 cup cold water
- 6 cups cooked noodles, warm

Directions

1. Place first seven ingredients in a crock pot; cover and cook on low 8 hours.
2. Remove pork shoulder and shred. Season with sea salt and black pepper.
3. Turn the crock pot to high and cook 10 more minutes. Stir in combined cornstarch and cold water, stirring often 2 to 3 minutes.

4. Return shredded pork to the crock pot and toss; serve over cooked noodles and enjoy.

Nutrition: Calories: 367 Fat: 28 g Carbs: 1 g Protein: 23 g

23. Teriyaki Pork with Tortillas

Preparation Time: 5 minutes

Cooking time: 8 hrs.

Servings: 6

Ingredients

- 1cup vegetable stock
- 1/4 cup dry red wine
- 1 pork shoulder roast, boneless
- 1 package (1.06 ounces) teriyaki marinade mix
- 2cloves garlic, minced
- 1 cup onion, chopped
- 1 teaspoon dried rosemary
- 1/2 teaspoon cumin seeds
- Sea salt, to taste
- Ground black pepper, to taste
- Red pepper flakes, crushed
- 6 flour tortillas

Directions

1. Add all of the ingredients, except tortillas, to the crock pot.
2. Cook on low heat setting approximately 8 hours or until the pork is falling-apart tender.
3. Next, cut cooked pork into shreds. Roll up in warm tortillas and enjoy!

Nutrition: Calories: 123 Fat: 15 g Carbs: 4 g Protein: 12 g

24. Pork Chops with Creamy Sauce

Preparation Time: 5 minutes

Cooking time: 5 hrs.

Servings46

Ingredients

- 4 loin pork chops, boneless
- Salt to taste
- Freshly ground black pepper, to taste
- 1/2 cup leeks, thinly sliced
- 1small rib celery, sliced
- 1 can (10 ounces) cream of celery soup
- 1/2 cup 2% reduced fat milk
- Cornbread, as garnish

Directions

1. Sprinkle pork with salt and freshly ground black pepper; add to the crock pot.
2. Place leeks and sliced celery on top.
3. Combine cream of celery soup with milk; whisk to combine. Pour the mixture into the crock pot.
4. Cover the crock pot with a lid and cook on low 4 to 5 hours. Serve with cornbread.

Nutrition: Calories: 156 Fat: 12 g Carbs: 3 g Protein: 21 g

25. Pork Chops with Apricot and Hoisin Sauce

Preparation Time: 5 minutes

Cooking time: 3 hrs.

Servings: 6

Ingredients

- 6 pork chops, boneless
- 1/2 teaspoon seasoned salt
- 1/2 teaspoon ground black pepper
- 1/2 teaspoon paprika
- 1/4 cup vegetable broth
- 1/2 cup apricot preserves
- 3 tablespoons hoisin sauce
- 1 tablespoon cornstarch

Directions

1. Sprinkle meat with salt, pepper and paprika; place in a crock pot; pour in vegetable broth.
2. Cover and cook on low heat setting about 3 hours; reserve pork chops.
3. To make the sauce, turn heat to high and cook 10 more minutes; add the rest of ingredients into the broth, stirring 2 to 3 minutes.
4. Serve warm over steamed vegetables.

Nutrition: Calories: 267 Fat: 11 g Carbs: 3 g Protein: 21 g

26. Pork Chops with Honey and Mustard

Preparation Time: 5 minutes

Cooking time: 4 hrs.

Servings: 4

Ingredients

- 4 loin pork chops, boneless
- 1/4 cup leeks, chopped
- 1/2 cup chicken broth
- 1/2 cup dry white wine
- 1/2 tablespoon cornstarch
- 1/2 tablespoons honey
- 1 tablespoons mustard
- 1 teaspoon grated ginger
- Salt, to taste
- Black pepper, to taste

Directions

1. Combine pork chops, leeks, chicken broth and white wine in a crock pot.
2. Cover and cook on low about 3 to 4 hours.
3. Remove pork chops from the crock pot and keep warm.
4. Add cornstarch, honey, mustard, ginger, salt and black pepper; continue cooking about 5 minutes. Serve warm.

Nutrition: Calories: 267 Fat: 11 g Carbs: 3 g Protein: 21 g

27. Smoked Pork with Prunes

Preparation Time: 5 minutes

Cooking time: 4 hrs.

Servings: 8

Ingredients

- 2 pounds pork loin, boneless and cubed
- 1cup prunes, pitted
- 1 1/2 cups vegetable broth
- 1/2 cup dry white wine
- 1 teaspoon lemon juice
- Salt, to taste
- Black pepper, to taste
- Smoked paprika, to taste
- 1/2tablespoons corn starch
- 1/4 cup cold water
- Liquid smoke, to taste
- 2cups cooked couscous, warm

Directions

1. Place all of the ingredients, except corn starch, water, liquid smoke and couscous, in a crock pot.
2. Cover and cook on low approximately 8 hours. Next, turn heat to high; cook about 10 minutes.
3. In a bowl, combine corn starch with cold water. Add this mixture and liquid smoke to the crock pot and stir constantly 2 to 3 minutes. Serve with couscous.

Nutrition: Calories: 476 Fat: 13 g Carbs: 5 g Protein: 12 g

28. Sweet Orange Smoked Ham

Preparation Time: 5 minutes

Cooking time: 3 hrs.

Servings: 10

Ingredients

- 3 pounds smoked ham, boneless
- 1/3 cup orange juice
- 1/4 cup honey
- 1 teaspoon allspice
- 1/2 teaspoon ground cinnamon
- 1 1/2 tablespoons corn starch
- 1/4 cup cold water
- 1/2 tablespoons dry sherry

Directions

1. Put all of the ingredients, except corn starch, water and sherry, into a crock pot.
2. Cover and cook on low until ham is tender or about 3 hours. Transfer prepared ham to a serving platter.
3. Measure 1 cup broth into skillet; heat to boiling; whisk in combined remaining ingredients about 1 minute.
4. Serve ham with sauce and enjoy!

Nutrition: Calories: 476 Fat: 13 g Carbs: 5 g Protein: 12 g

29. Sherry Chicken with Mashed Potatoes

Preparation Time: 5 minutes

Cooking time: 4 hrs.

Servings: 4

Ingredients

- For the Sherry Chicken:
- 1/4 cup dry sherry
- 1cup raisins
- 4 medium-sized chicken breasts
- 1 tart cooking apple, peeled and chopped
- 1 sweet onion, sliced
- 1 cup chicken broth
- Salt and pepper, to taste
- 2pounds Idaho potatoes, peeled and cooked
- 1/4 sour cream
- 1/3 cup whole milk
- 1/2tablespoons butter
- 1 teaspoon sea salt
- 1/4 teaspoon black pepper
- 1/4 teaspoon cayenne pepper

Directions

1. In a crock pot, place all of the ingredients for the sherry chicken; cover and cook on high until chicken breasts are tender or 3 to 4 hours.

2. Meanwhile, beat potatoes, adding sour cream, milk, and butter; beat until smooth and uniform.
3. Season with spices and serve on the side with sherry chicken.

Nutrition: Calories: 154 Fat: 12 g Carbs: 3 g Protein: 15 g

SNACKS RECIPES

30. Nectarines with Dried Cloves

Preparation Time: 5 Minutes

Cooking Time: 50 minutes

Servings: 4

Ingredients:

- 4 dried cloves, whole
- 2lb.s. nectarine, cubed
- 1/4cup agave sugar, reserve for garnish
- 1/16tsp. cinnamon powder
- 2cups water

Directions:

1. Combine dried cloves, nectarine, water, cinnamon powder, and agave sugar into the Instant Pot Pressure Cooker.
2. Lock the lid in place. Press the high pressure and cook for 5 minutes.
3. When the beep sounds, Choose the Quick Pressure Release. This will depressurize for 7 minutes. Remove the lid. Discard dried cloves.
4. To serve, ladle just the right amount into dessert bowls. Sprinkle agave sugar.

Nutrition: Calories 267 Fat 23 Fiber 19 Carbs 5 Protein 21

31. Chocolate Raspberry Parfait

Preparation Time: 5 Minutes

Cooking Time: 50 minutes

Servings: 2

Ingredients:

- Raspberry chia seeds
- 3Tbsp. chia seeds
- 1/2cup almond milk, unsweetened
- 1/4tsp. sugar
- 1cup frozen raspberries, reserve some for garnish
- 1/8tsp. lemon juice, freshly squeezed
- Chocolate tapioca
- 1/2Tbsp. Dutch cocoa powder
- 1/8cup seed tapioca, picked over
- 1cup almond milk, unsweetened
- 1cup water
- 4 squares dark chocolate, chopped, reserve some for garnish

Directions

1. For the raspberry chia seeds, combine chia seeds, almond milk, sugar, raspberries, and lemon juice in a bowl. Mix well. Mash berries. Seal with saran wrap. Place inside the fridge until ready to use.
2. For the chocolate tapioca, put together cocoa powder, tapioca, almond milk, water, and dark chocolate into the crockpot. Stir.

3. Lock the lid in place. Press the high pressure and cook for 8 minutes.
4. When the beep sounds, Choose Natural Pressure Release. Depressurizing would take 20 minutes. Remove the lid.
5. To serve, spoon in half portions of chocolate tapioca in heat-proof glass. Put just the right amount of raspberry-chia mixture on top. Garnish with whole raspberries and chopped chocolate.

Nutrition: Calories 321 Fat 22 Fiber 11 Carbs 4 Protein 26

32. Patbingsu – In Moderation

Preparation Time: 5 Minutes

Cooking Time: 55 minutes

Servings: 6

Ingredients:

- 1/4cup dried red kidney beans, picked over
- 1cup dried Adzuki beans, picked over
- 1/4cup dried pinto beans, picked over
- 6cups water
- 1/2Tbsp. coconut oil
- 1cup brown sugar
- 1/16tsp. green tea powder
- 1/2cup loosely packed shaved ice, per person, prepare this only when about to serve
- 1/4cup almond milk, chilled

Directions:

1. For the bean base, place red kidney beans, adzuki beans, pinto beans, water, and coconut oil into the Instant Pot Pressure Cooker. Stir well.
2. Lock the lid in place. Press the high pressure and cook for 30 minutes.
3. When the beep sounds, Choose Natural Pressure Release. Depressurizing would take 20 minutes. Remove the lid.
4. Drain beans and reserve at least half of the cooking liquid. Put back into the crockpot.

5. Press the "Sauté" button. Stir in brown sugar. Turn off the machine immediately. Let it for 15 minutes or until it thickens.
6. To serve, place shaved ice into bowls. Spoon just the right amount of bean base. Garnish with green tea powder. Drizzle in almond milk. Serve.

Nutrition: Calories 216 Fat 32 Fiber 11 Carbs 4.9 Protein 26

VEGETABLE RECIPES

33. Cheese Stuffed Spaghetti Squash

Preparation time: 15 minutes

Cooking time: 50 to 60 minutes

Servings: 4

Ingredients:

- ½ pound (227 g) spaghetti squash, halved, scoop out seeds
- teaspoon olive oil
- ½ cup Mozzarella cheese, shredded
- ½ cup cream cheese
- ½ cup full-fat Greek yogurt
- 2 eggs
- 1 garlic clove, minced
- ½ teaspoon cumin
- ½ teaspoon basil ½ teaspoon mint
- Sea salt and ground black pepper, to taste

Directions:

1. Place the squash halves in a baking pan; drizzle the insides of each squash half with olive oil.
2. Bake in the preheated oven at 370ºF (188ºC) for 45 to 50 minutes or until the interiors are easily pierced through with a fork

3. Now, scrape out the spaghetti squash "noodles" from the skin in a mixing bowl. Add the remaining ingredients and mix to combine well.//
4. Carefully fill each of the squash half with the cheese mixture. Bake at 350ºF (180ºC) for 5 to 10 minutes, until the cheese is bubbling and golden brown. Bon appétit!

Nutrition: calories: 220 fat: 17.6g protein: 9.0g carbs: 6.8g net carbs: 5.9g fiber: 0.9g

34. Cottage Kale Stir-Fry

Preparation time: 10 minutes

Cooking time: 10 minutes

Servings: 3

Ingredients:

- ½ tablespoon olive oil
- 1 teaspoon fresh garlic, chopped
- 9 ounces (255 g) kale, torn into pieces
- ½ cup Cottage cheese, creamed
- ½ teaspoon sea salt

Directions:

1. Heat the olive oil in a saucepan over a moderate flame. Now, cook the garlic until just tender and aromatic.
2. Then, stir in the kale and continue to cook for about 10 minutes until all liquid evaporates.
3. Fold in the Cottage cheese and salt; stir until everything is heated through. Enjoy!

Nutrition: calories: 94 fat: 4.5g protein: 7.0g carbs: 6.2g net carbs: 3.5g fiber: 2.7g

35. Herbed Eggplant and Kale Bake

Preparation time: 20 minutes

Cooking time: 40 minutes

Servings: 6

Ingredients:

- 1 (¾-pound / 340-g) eggplant, cut into ½-inch slices
- 1 tablespoon olive oil
- 1 tablespoon butter, melted
- 8 ounces (227 g) kale leaves, torn into pieces
- 14 ounces (397 g) garlic-and-tomato pasta sauce, without sugar
- 1/3 cup cream cheese
- 1 cup Asiago cheese, shredded
- ½ cup Gorgonzola cheese, grated
- 2 tablespoons ketchup, without sugar
- 1 teaspoon hot pepper
- 1 teaspoon basil
- 1 teaspoon oregano
- ½ teaspoon rosemary

Directions:

1. Place the eggplant slices in a colander and sprinkle them with salt. Allow it to sit for 2 hours. Wipe the eggplant slices with paper towels.
2. Brush the eggplant slices with olive oil; cook in a cast-iron grill pan until nicely browned on both sides, about 5 minutes.

3. Melt the butter in a pan over medium flame. Now, cook the kale leaves until wilted. In a mixing bowl, combine the three types of cheese.
4. Transfer the grilled eggplant slices to a lightly greased baking dish. Top with the kale. Then, add a layer of ½ of cheese blend.
5. Pour the tomato sauce over the cheese layer. Top with the remaining cheese mixture. Sprinkle with seasoning.
6. Bake in the preheated oven at 350ºF (180ºC) until cheese is bubbling and golden brown, about 35 minutes. Bon appétit!

Nutrition: calories: 231 fat: 18.6g protein: 10.5g carbs: 6.7g net carbs: 4.3g fiber: 2.4g

POULTRY RECIPES

36. Chicken Meatloaf Cups with Pancetta

Preparation Time: 15 minutes

Cooking Time: 30 minutes

Servings: 6

Ingredients:

- 2tbsp. onion, chopped
- 1tsp. garlic, minced
- 1-pound ground chicken
- 2ounces cooked pancetta, chopped
- 1egg, beaten
- 1tsp. mustard
- Salt and black pepper, to taste
- 1/2tsp. crushed red pepper flakes
- 1tsp. dried basil
- 1/2tsp. dried oregano
- 4 ounces cheddar cheese, cubed

Directions:

1. In a mixing bowl, mix mustard, onion, ground turkey, egg, bacon, and garlic. Season with oregano, red pepper, black pepper, basil, and salt.
2. Split the mixture into muffin cups—lower one cube of cheddar cheese into each meatloaf cup.
3. Close the top to cover the cheese.

4. Bake in the oven at 345ºF for 20 minutes, or until the meatloaf cups become golden brown.

Nutrition: Calories: 231 Fat: 10.4g Fiber: 5.1g Carbohydrates: 3.9 g Protein: 11.4g

37. Turkey Wing Curry

Preparation time: 15 minutes

Cooking time: 55 minutes

Servings: 4

Ingredients:

- 3 teaspoons sesame oil
- 1 pound (454 g) turkey wings, boneless and chopped
- 2 cloves garlic, finely chopped
- 1 small-sized red chili pepper, minced
- ½ teaspoon turmeric powder
- ½ teaspoon ginger powder
- 1 teaspoon red curry paste
- 1 cup unsweetened coconut milk, preferably homemade
- ½ cup water
- ½ cup turkey consommé
- Kosher salt and ground black pepper, to taste

Directions:

1. Heat sesame oil in a sauté pan. Add the turkey and cook until it is light brown about 7 minutes.
2. Add garlic, chili pepper, turmeric powder, ginger powder, and curry paste and cook for 3 minutes longer.
3. Add the milk, water, and consommé. Season with salt and black pepper. Cook for 45 minutes over medium heat. Bon appétit!

Nutrition: calories: 296 Fat: 19.6g protein: 25.6g carbs: 3.0g net carbs: 3.0g fiber: 0g

38. Double-Cheese Ranch Chicken

Preparation time: 15 minutes

Cooking time: 20 minutes

Servings: 4

Ingredients:

- 2 chicken breasts
- 2 tablespoons butter, melted
- 1 teaspoon salt
- ½ teaspoon garlic powder
- ½ teaspoon cayenne pepper
- ½ teaspoon black peppercorns, crushed
- ½ tablespoon ranch seasoning mix
- 4 ounces (113 g) Ricotta cheese, room temperature
- ½ cup Monterey-Jack cheese, grated
- 4 slices bacon, chopped
- ¼ cup scallions, chopped

Directions:

1. Start by preheating your oven to 370ºF (188ºC).
2. Drizzle the chicken with melted butter. Rub the chicken with salt, garlic powder, cayenne pepper, black pepper, and ranch seasoning mix.
3. Heat a cast iron skillet over medium heat. Cook the chicken for 3 to 5 minutes per side. Transfer the chicken to a lightly greased baking dish.
4. Add cheese and bacon. Bake about 12 minutes. Top with scallions just before serving. Bon appétit!

Nutrition: calories: 290 Fat: 19.3g protein: 25.1g carbs: 2.5g net carbs: 2.5g fiber: 0g

39. Turkey and Canadian Bacon Pizza

Preparation time: 10 minutes

Cooking time: 32minutes

Servings: 4

Ingredients:

- ½ pound (227 g) ground turkey
- ½ cup Parmesan cheese, freshly grated
- ½ cup Mozzarella cheese, grated
- Salt and ground black pepper, to taste
- 1bell pepper, sliced
- 2slices Canadian bacon, chopped
- 1tomato, chopped
- 1teaspoon oregano
- ½ teaspoon basil

Directions:

1. In mixing bowl, thoroughly combine the ground turkey, cheese, salt, and black pepper.
2. Then, press the cheese-chicken mixture into a parchment-lined baking pan. Bake in the preheated oven, at 390ºF (199ºC) for 22minutes.
3. Add bell pepper, bacon, tomato, oregano, and basil. Bake an additional 10 minutes and serve warm. Bon appétit!

Nutrition: calories: 361 Fat: 22.6g protein: 32.5g carbs: 5.8g net carbs: 5.2g fiber: 0.6g

FISH AND SEAFOOD RECIPES

40. Coconut Mussels

Preparation Time: 10 minutes

Cooking Time: 10-15 minutes

Servings: 4

Ingredients:

- 2tablespoons coconut oil
- 1/2sweet onion, chopped
- 2teaspoons minced garlic
- 1teaspoon grated fresh ginger
- 1/2teaspoon turmeric
- 1cup of coconut milk
- Juice of 1lime
- 11/2pounds fresh mussels, scrubbed and debearded
- 1scallion, finely chopped
- 2tablespoons chopped fresh cilantro
- 1tablespoon chopped fresh thyme

Directions:

1. Sauté the aromatics.
2. In a pot, warm the coconut oil. Add the onion, garlic, ginger, and turmeric and sauté until they've softened about 3 minutes.
3. Add the liquid. Stir in the coconut milk and lime juice and bring the mixture to a boil.

4. Steam the mussels.
5. Add the mussels to the skillet, cover, and steam until the shells are open, about 10 minutes.
6. Take the skillet off the heat and throw out any unopened mussels.
7. Add the herbs. Stir in the scallion, cilantro, and thyme.
8. Serve. Divide the mussels and the sauce between four bowls and serve them immediately.

Nutrition: Calories: 321 Fat: 11.1g Fiber: 9g Carbohydrates: 1.2g Protein: 1.4g

41. Italian Style Halibut Packets

Preparation Time: 10 minutes

Cooking Time: 20 minutes

Servings: 4

Ingredients:

- 2cups cauliflower florets
- 1cup roasted red pepper strips
- 1/2cup sliced sun-dried tomatoes
- 4 (4-ounce) halibut fillets
- 1/4 cup chopped fresh basil
- Juice of 1lemon
- 1/4 cup good-quality olive oil
- Sea salt, for seasoning
- Freshly ground black pepper, for seasoning

Directions:

1. Preheat the oven. Set the oven temperature to 400°F.
2. Make the packets.
3. Divide the cauliflower, red pepper strips, and sun-dried tomato between the four pieces of foil, placing the vegetables in the middle of each piece.
4. Top each pile with one halibut fillet, and top each fillet with equal amounts of the basil, lemon juice, and olive oil.
5. Fold and crimp the foil to form sealed packets of fish and vegetables and place them on the baking sheet.

6. Bake. Bake the packets for about 20 minutes, until the fish flakes with a fork.
7. Be careful of the steam when you open the packet!
8. Serve. Transfer the vegetables and halibut to four plates, season with salt and pepper, and serve immediately.

Nutrition: Calories: 313 Fat: 14.1g Fiber: 10.4g Carbohydrates: 3.2g Protein: 15.4g

42. Hazelnut Haddock Bake

Preparation time: 15 minutes

Cooking time: 25 minutes

Servings: 4

Ingredients:

- 1tablespoon butter
- 1shallot, sliced
- 1pound (454 g) haddock fillet
- 2eggs, hard-boiled, chopped
- ½ cup water
- 3 tablespoons hazelnut flour
- 2cups sour cream
- 1tablespoon parsley, chopped
- ½ cup pork rinds, crushed
- 1cup Mozzarella cheese, grated
- Salt and black pepper to taste

Directions:

1. Melt butter in a saucepan over medium heat and sauté the shallots for about 3 minutes.
2. Reduce the heat to low and stir the hazelnut flour into it to form a roux. Cook the roux to be golden brown and stir in the sour cream until the mixture is smooth. Season with salt and pepper, and stir in the parsley.
3. Spread the haddock fillet in a greased baking dish, sprinkle the eggs on top, and spoon the sauce over. In a

bowl, mix the pork rinds with the Mozzarella cheese, and sprinkle it over the sauce.

4. Bake in the oven for 20 minutes at 370ºF (188ºC) until the top is golden and the sauce and cheese are bubbly.

Nutrition: calories: 786 Fat: 56.9g Protein: 64.9g Carbs: 9.5g net carbs: 8.4g Fiber: 1.1g

43. Coconut and Pecorino Fried Shrimp

Preparation time: 15 minutes

Cooking time: 10 minutes

Servings: 4

Ingredients:

- 2 teaspoons coconut flour
- 2 tablespoons grated Pecorino cheese
- 1 egg, beaten in a bowl
- ¼ teaspoon curry powder
- 1 pound (454 g) shrimp, shelled
- 3 tablespoons coconut oil
- Salt to taste
- Sauce:
- 2 tablespoons butter
- 2 tablespoons cilantro leaves, chopped
- ½ onion, diced
- ½ cup coconut cream
- ½ ounce (14 g) Paneer cheese, grated

Directions:

1. Combine coconut flour, Pecorino cheese, curry powder, and salt in a bowl.
2. Melt the coconut oil in a skillet over medium heat. Dip the shrimp in the egg first, and then coat with the dry mixture. Fry until golden and crispy, about 5 minutes.

3. In another skillet, melt the butter. Add onion and cook for 3 minutes. Add curry and cilantro and cook for 30 seconds. Stir in coconut cream and Paneer cheese and cook until thickened. Add the shrimp and coat well. Serve warm.

Nutrition: calories: 740 Fat: 63.8g Protein: 34.2g Carbs: 5.2g net carbs: 4.2g Fiber: 1.0g

44. Greek Tilapia with Tomatoes and Olives

Preparation time: 10 minutes

Cooking time: 15 minutes

Servings: 4

Ingredients:

- 4 tilapia fillets
- 2 garlic cloves, minced
- 2 teaspoons oregano
- 14 ounces (397 g) tomatoes, diced
- 1 tablespoon olive oil
- ½ red onion, chopped
- 2 tablespoons parsley
- ¼ cup kalamata olives

Directions:

1. Heat olive oil in a skillet over medium heat, and cook onion, garlic, and oregano for 3 minutes. Stir in tomatoes and bring the mixture to a boil. Reduce the heat and simmer, for 5 minutes. Add olives and tilapia. Cook, for about 8 minutes. Serve the tilapia with the tomato sauce.

Nutrition: calories: 183 Fat: 15.0g Protein: 22.9g Carbs: 7.9g net carbs: 6.2g Fiber: 1.7g

SALAD RECIPES

45. Charred Broccoli and Sardine Salad

Preparation time: 5 minutes

Cooking time: 5 minutes

Servings: 4

Ingredients:

- 1pound (454 g) broccoli florets
- ½ white onion, thinly sliced
- 2(4-ounce / 113-g) cans sardines in oil, drained
- 2tablespoons fresh lime juice
- 1teaspoon stone-ground mustard

Directions:

1. Heat a lightly greased cast-iron skillet over medium-high heat. Cook the broccoli florets for 5 to 6 minutes until charred; work in batches.
2. In salad bowls, place the charred broccoli with onion and sardines. Toss with the lime juice and mustard. Serve at room temperature. Bon appétit!

Nutrition: calories: 160 fat: 7.2g protein: 17.6g carbs: 5.6g net carbs: 2.6g fiber: 3.0g

46. Zucchini and Bell Pepper Slaw

Preparation time: 15 minutes

Cooking time: 0 minutes

Servings: 3

Ingredients:

- 1zucchini, shredded
- 1yellow bell pepper, sliced
- 1red onion, thinly sliced
- 2tablespoons extra-virgin olive oil
- 1tablespoon balsamic vinegar
- 1teaspoon Dijon mustard
- ¼ teaspoon cumin seeds
- ¼ teaspoon ground black pepper
- Sea salt, to taste

Directions:

1. Thoroughly combine all ingredients in a salad bowl.
2. Refrigerate for 1hour before serving or serve right away. Enjoy!

Nutrition: calories: 97 fat: 9.5g protein: 0.8g carbs: 2.7g net carbs: 2.4g fiber: 0.3g

DESSERT

47. Delicious Peach Crisp

Preparation Time: 10 minutes

Cooking Time: 45 minutes

Serve: 8

Ingredients:

- 8 cups can peach, sliced
- 1/2cup butter, cubed
- 1/2cup brown sugar
- 1/2cup all-purpose flour
- 11/2cups rolled oats
- 2tbsp. cornstarch
- 1/2cup sugar

Directions:

1. Add peaches, cornstarch, and sugar into the cooking pot and stir well.
2. Mix together butter, brown sugar, flour, and oats and sprinkle over peaches.
3. Cover instant pot aura with lid.
4. Select Bake mode and set the temperature to 350 F and time for 30-45 minutes.
5. Serve with ice cream

Nutrition: Calories 478, Fat 12, Carbs 3.7, Protein 3

48. Gingerbread Pudding Cake

Preparation Time: 10 minutes

Cooking Time: 2hours 30 minutes

Serve: 6

Ingredients:

- 1egg
- 11/4 cups whole wheat flour
- 1/8 tsp. ground nutmeg
- 1/2tsp. ground ginger
- 1/2tsp. ground cinnamon
- 3/4 tsp. baking soda
- 1cup of water
- 1/2cup molasses
- 1tsp. vanilla
- 1/4 cup sugar
- 1/4 cup butter, softened
- 1/4 tsp. salt

Directions:

1. In a bowl, beat sugar and butter until combined. Add egg and beat until combined.
2. Add water, molasses, and vanilla and beat until well combined.
3. Add flour, nutmeg, ginger, cinnamon, baking soda, and salt and stir until combined.
4. Pour batter into the cooking pot.
5. Cover instant pot aura with lid.

6. Select slow cook mode and cook on HIGH for 21/2hours.
7. Serve with vanilla ice-cream.

Nutrition: Calories 278, Fat 8, Carbs 4.9, Protein 3

49. Healthy Blueberry Cobbler

Preparation Time: 10 minutes

Cooking Time: 2hours 30 minutes

Serve: 6

Ingredients:

- 2 1/4 cups all-purpose flour
- 4 cups blueberries
- 8 tbsp. butter, melted
- 1tsp. cinnamon
- 1tbsp. cornstarch
- 3 1/2tsp. baking powder
- 1 1/4 cups sugar
- 1tsp. salt

Directions:

1. Add blueberries into the cooking pot.
2. Mix together flour, cinnamon, cornstarch, baking powder, sugar, and salt and sprinkle over blueberries evenly.
3. Pour melted butter over flour mixture evenly.
4. Cover instant pot aura with lid.
5. Select slow cook mode and cook on LOW for 2 1/2hours.
6. Serve with vanilla ice-cream.

Nutrition: Calories 570, Fat 16, Carbs 1.3, Protein 5

50. Easy Peach Cobbler

Preparation Time: 10 minutes

Cooking Time: 3 hours

Serve: 6

Ingredients:

- 1/2cup butter, cut into pieces
- 1box cake mix
- 30 oz. can sliced peaches in syrup

Directions:

1. Add sliced peaches with syrup into the cooking pot.
2. Sprinkle cake mix on top of sliced peaches.
3. Spread butter pieces on top of the cake mix.
4. Cover instant pot aura with lid.
5. Select slow cook mode and cook on HIGH for 3 hours.
6. Serve with vanilla ice-cream.

Nutrition: Calories 602, Fat 12, Carbs 5, Protein 11

KETO MEDITERRANEAN RECIPES

51. Vanilla Frozen Yogurt

Servings: 8

Preparation time: 35 minutes; Cooking Time:0 minute;

NUTRITION:Calories: 122 Cal, Carbs: 2.7 g, Fat: 11.4 g, Protein: 3.2 g, Fiber: 0 g.

INGREDIENTS:
- 4 tablespoons monk fruit sweetener, grounded
- 2 teaspoons vanilla extract, unsweetened
- 1 tablespoon lemon juice
- 1 tablespoon olive oil
- 3 cups chilled plain yogurt, full fat

DIRECTIONS:
1. Place all the ingredients in a blender and pulse for 1 to 2 minutes or until blended and creamy.
2. Spoon this mixture into a freezer safe container, cover with its lid and chill for 30 minutes or until soft but firm ice cream comes together.

3. Serve straightaway.

52. Chia Berry Yogurt Parfaits

Servings: 4

Preparation time: 10 minutes; Cooking Time:0 minutes;

NUTRITION: Calories: 319 Cal, Carbs: 15.3 g, Fat: 25.1 g, Protein: 12.1 g, Fiber: 7.6 g.

INGREDIENTS:

- 1 cup mixed berries, frozen
- 1/3 cup flaked coconut, toasted
- 1/3 cup chia seeds
- 2 tablespoons sunflower seeds
- 2 tablespoons pumpkin seeds
- 1 tablespoon Erythritol
- 1/4 teaspoon ground cinnamon
- 1/2 teaspoon vanilla extract, unsweetened
- 1/2 cup coconut cream, full-fat
- 1 cup Greek yogurt
- 2/3 cup water

DIRECTIONS:

1. Stir together chia seeds, Erythritol, cinnamon, vanilla, coconut cream, and water until well combined and then spoon in a bottom of a serving bowl.

2. Mix berries and yogurt with a fork until crushed and smooth paste form and then spoon this mixture in an even layer on top of the chia seed layer.
3. Stir together sunflower seeds, pumpkin seeds and coconut flakes and top this mixture on the berries-yogurt layer.
4. Serve straightaway.

53. Lemon Meringue Cookies

Servings: 15

Preparation time: 2 hours and 10 minutes; Cooking Time: 1 hour;

NUTRITION: Calories: 2 Cal, Carbs: 0 g, Fat: 0 g, Protein: 0.5 g, Fiber: 0 g.

INGREDIENTS:
- 1/4 cup Erythritol
- 1/2 tablespoon lemon zest
- 1/2 teaspoon lemon juice
- 2 egg whites, pasture-raised

DIRECTIONS:
1. Set oven to 200 degrees F and let preheat.
2. In the meantime, place egg whites in a large bowl and blend using a stick blender until stiff peaks forms.
3. Then beat in lemon juice until hard peaks forms and then beat in sweetener, 1 tablespoon at a time, until well mixed and slowly beat in lemon zest.
4. Spoon this mixture into a piping bag and form cookies on a baking sheet, lined with a parchment sheet.

5. Place the baking sheet into the heated oven and bake for 1 hour, then switch off the oven and let cookies rest in oven for 1 to 2 hours until cool completely.
6. Serve straightaway.

54. Strawberry Cheesecake Jars

Servings: 4

Preparation time: 1 hour and 10 minutes; Cooking Time: 0 minutes;

NUTRITION: Calories: 375 Cal, Carbs: 6.9 g, Fat: 36.5 g, Protein: 4.3 g, Fiber: 1.2 g.

INGREDIENTS:

- 1 cup and 1 tablespoon strawberry and basil chia jam
- 1/4 cup powdered Erythritol
- 1 teaspoon lemon zest
- 1/2 teaspoon vanilla extract, unsweetened
- 1 tablespoon lemon juice
- 1 cup coconut cream, full-fat
- 1 cup cream cheese, full-fat
- 1/2 cup sour cream, full-fat

DIRECTIONS:

1. Beat together lemon zest, vanilla, coconut cream, and cream cheese with a stick blender until smooth.
2. Divide this mixture evenly into 6 jars, each about 4-ounce, then top with 2 tablespoons of strawberry and basil chia jam.

3. Place these jars in the refrigerator for 1 hour or until chilled and then serve.

55. Tuscan Garlic Chicken

Servings: 4

Preparation time: 5 minutes; Cooking Time: 10 minutes;

NUTRITION: Calories: 487.7 Cal, Carbs: 7.3 g, Fat: 35.8 g, Protein: 33.8 g, Fiber: 1.2 g.

INGREDIENTS:

- 1½ pounds skinless pasture-raised chicken breasts, thinly sliced
- 1 cup fresh spinach, chopped
- ½ cup sun-dried tomatoes
- 1 teaspoon garlic powder
- 1 teaspoon Italian seasoning
- 2 tablespoons olive oil
- ½ cup parmesan cheese, full-fat
- 1 cup heavy cream, full-fat
- ½ cup chicken broth, pasture-raised

DIRECTIONS:

1. Place a large skillet over high heat, add oil and when hot, add chicken breast pieces.
2. Cook for 3 to 5 minutes or until nicely golden brown on each side and then transfer chicken pieces to a plate.

3. Return pan over medium-high heat, add remaining ingredients except for spinach and tomatoes and whisk well.
4. Cook for 1 to 2 minutes or until mixture starts to thicken, then add spinach and tomatoes and simmer for 3 minutes or until spinach leaves wilt.
5. Return chicken to pan and stir well.
6. Serve when ready.

56. Garlic & Rosemary Lamb Lollipops

Servings: 2

Preparation time: 10 minutes; Cooking Time: 10 minutes;

NUTRITION: Calories: 171.5 Cal, Carbs: 0.4 g, Fat: 7.8 g, Protein: 23.2 g, Fiber: 0.1 g.

INGREDIENTS:
- 8 lamb lollipops, pastured
- 2 tablespoons rosemary leaves
- 1 teaspoon minced garlic
- 1 teaspoon salt
- ¾ teaspoon cracked black pepper
- 3 tablespoons olive oil

DIRECTIONS:
1. Season lamb with salt and black pepper on each side and then sprinkle with 1 tablespoon rosemary leaves.
2. Place a large skillet pan over medium-high heat, add oil and when hot, add remaining rosemary leaves and garlic and then lamb lollipops.
3. Cook lamb lollipops for 5 minutes per side until seared.
4. Serve immediately.

57. Greek Chicken

Servings: 4

Preparation time: 1 hour and 10 minutes; Cooking Time:16 minutes;

NUTRITION: Calories: 261 Cal, Carbs: 1.8 g, Fat: 19 g, Protein: 21 g, Fiber: 1.5 g.

INGREDIENTS:

- 4 skinless chicken breasts, pasture-raised
- 1 cup chopped cherry tomatoes
- 1/3 cup sliced Kalamata olives
- 2 teaspoons minced garlic
- 3 tablespoons chopped oregano, fresh
- 1 teaspoon salt
- ¾ teaspoon cracked black pepper
- 1/2 cup and 2 tablespoons olive oil
- 1/2 cup lemon juice
- 1/2 cup crumbled Feta cheese, full-fat

DIRECTIONS:

1. Score top of each chicken breast in crisscross and place in a re-sealable plastic bag.

2. Whisk together garlic, oregano, lemon juice, and ½ cup olive oil until combined, reserve ¼ cup of this mixture and pour remaining mixture into a plastic bag containing chicken pieces.
3. Seal the bag, turn it upside until chicken pieces are well coated and let marinate in the refrigerator for 1 hour.
4. When ready to cook, take out the chicken from the refrigerator and let rest at room temperature.
5. In the meantime, place reserved marinade in a bowl, add tomatoes, olives, and cheese and toss until well coated.
6. Place a large skillet pan over medium-high heat, add 1 tablespoon oil and when hot, add marinated chicken in a single layer, scored side down.
7. Cook for 4 minutes per side or until chicken is no longer pink, then season with salt and black and transfer to a plate.
8. Add remaining oil to the pan and cook remaining chicken in the same manner.
9. Top chicken with tomato-olives-feta topping and serve.

58. Lemon Chicken

Servings: 4

Preparation time: 10 minutes; Cooking Time: 15 minutes;

NUTRITION: Calories: 282 Cal, Carbs: 5 g, Fat: 18 g, Protein: 26 g, Fiber: 1 g.

INGREDIENTS:

- 1-pound skinless pasture-raised chicken breast, cut into 4 slices
- 1 cup cherry tomatoes
- 1/2 cup white onions, peeled and cut into 1/4-inch slices
- 1 teaspoon minced garlic
- 1/2 teaspoon onion powder
- 1/2 teaspoon garlic powder
- 1 teaspoon salt
- 1/4 teaspoon cracked black pepper, freshly ground
- 1/2 teaspoon paprika
- 2 sprigs of thyme
- 3 sprigs of rosemary
- 1 1/2 teaspoons ground cumin
- 1/2 teaspoon ground coriander
- 1/4 cup olive oil
- 3 tablespoons lemon juice

DIRECTIONS:

1. Stir together onion powder, garlic powder, salt, black pepper, paprika, cumin and coriander in a bowl.
2. Sprinkle ½ teaspoon of this spice mix on each side of the chicken piece.
3. Place a large skillet pan over medium-high heat, add oil and when hot, add onion and garlic.
4. Cook for 2 minutes, move to the side and then add tomatoes to the pan.
5. Cook tomatoes for 3 minutes and then transfer onion and tomatoes to a bowl.
6. Add thyme and rosemary sprigs to skillet pan, then add seasoned chicken to the pan and cook for 4 to 5 minutes per side or until chicken is nicely browned.
7. Then remove the pan from heat, drizzle with lemon juice, top with onion and tomatoes and serve.

59. Chicken Pesto Meatballs

Servings: 20

Preparation time: 10 minutes; Cooking Time:20 minutes;

NUTRITION: Calories: 424 Cal, Carbs: 6.2 g, Fat: 32.9 g, Protein: 27.3 g, Fiber: 1.9 g.

INGREDIENTS:

- 1-pound ground chicken, pasture-raised
- 1 small red onion, peeled and chopped
- 1/2 cup almond flour
- 1/2 teaspoon sea salt
- 1/2 cup basil pesto, divided
- 1 egg, pasture-raised

DIRECTIONS:

1. Set oven to 375 degrees F and let preheat.
2. In the meantime, place chicken in a bowl, add onion, flour, salt, ¼ cup pesto, and egg and stir until well combined.
3. Shape this mixture into 16 meatballs and place onto a baking sheet, greased with olive oil.

4. Place the baking sheet into the heated oven and bake for 20 minutes or until nicely golden brown and cooked through.
5. When done, transfer meatballs to a serving plate, top with remaining pesto and serve.

60. Parmesan Chicken

Servings: 6

Preparation time: 10 minutes; Cooking Time: 30 minutes; Total time: 40 minutes

NUTRITION: Calories: 454 Cal, Carbs: 9.1 g, Fat: 24.8 g, Protein: 49.4 g, Fiber: 7.6 g.

INGREDIENTS:

- 6 skinless chicken breasts, pasture-raised
- 1/2 teaspoon garlic powder
- 1/2 teaspoon sea salt
- 1/2 teaspoon cracked black pepper
- 1/2 teaspoon dried oregano
- 1/2 cup and 1 tablespoon mayonnaise, full-fat
- 2/3 cup grated Parmesan cheese, full-fat
- 3/4 cup and 1 tablespoon coconut flakes, dried

DIRECTIONS:

1. Set oven to 430 degrees F and let preheat.
2. In the meantime, stir together garlic powder, garlic powder, salt, black pepper, oregano, coconut flakes and cheese in a bowl.
3. Place mayonnaise in another bowl.

4. Working on one chicken piece at a time, first season with salt, then coat with mayonnaise and cover evenly with flake mixture.
5. Place coated chicken breasts on a baking tray, lined with parchment sheet and place into the heated oven.
6. Bake for 30 minutes or until top is nicely browned and cooked through.
7. When done, slice chicken or serve straight away.

CPSIA information can be obtained
at www.ICGtesting.com
Printed in the USA
LVHW020951160721
692882LV00023B/1650